I0702263

MENOPAUSE DIET

FOR

WEIGHT LOSS

Women Athletes Guide To Hormone Balance

And 30-Day Exercise Plan To Burn Fat

DR. MINDY ANDERSON

Copyright © Dr, Mindy Anderson, 2023.

All rights reserved. No part of this publication may be reproduced, distributed, or transmitted in any form or by any means, including photocopying, recording, or other electronic or mechanical methods, without the prior written permission of the publisher, except in the case of brief quotations embodied in critical reviews and certain other noncommercial uses permitted by copyright law.

BONUS

EXERCISE JOURNAL ON THIS PAPERBACK VERSION

TABLE OF COTENTS

INTRODUCTION

Emily is a 47 years old lady who had always been an active and fit woman, but when she hit her late forties, she noticed some changes in her body that made her feel uncomfortable and insecure.

She started to gain weight, especially around her belly, and she felt hot flashes, mood swings, and insomnia. She knew these were signs of menopause, but she didn't want to accept them as inevitable.

She wanted to find a way to keep her health and vitality and to feel good about herself again.

That's when she discovered the Menopause Explains Weight Loss Guide, a book that changed her life.

This book explains how hormonal changes during menopause affect metabolism, appetite, and fat distribution, and how certain foods can help balance hormones, reduce inflammation, and prevent weight gain.

Emily decided to give the menopause diet for weight loss guide a try, and she was amazed by the results. Within a few weeks, she noticed that her weight stabilized, her belly fat reduced, and her energy levels increased.

She also felt fewer hot flashes, calmer, and more rested. She felt like she had regained control over her body and her life.

The menopause diet for weight loss guide was best for Emily, An era of transformation.

How she learned to embrace the changes in her body and to use them as an opportunity to improve her health and happiness.

A story of how she became a confident and radiant woman who enjoyed every stage of her life.

CHAPTER 1: UNDERSTANDING MENOPAUSE AND HORMONAL CHANGES

Menopause is a natural biological process that marks the end of a woman's reproductive years. It typically occurs in the late 40s or early 50s, although the exact timing can vary for each individual.

This transitional phase is characterized by the cessation of menstrual cycles, and it brings about a series of hormonal changes that have profound effects on a woman's body.

One of the primary contributors to menopause is the decline in the production of estrogen and progesterone, two key hormones that play crucial roles in the menstrual cycle and overall reproductive health.

As the ovaries gradually produce less of these hormones, the body undergoes various adjustments, leading to both physical and emotional changes.

This transition is often accompanied by a range of symptoms, including hot flashes, night sweats, and mood swings.

The fluctuating hormone levels can also impact the health of tissues in the reproductive and urinary tracts, leading to changes in vaginal health and an increased risk of urinary tract infections.

Beyond the reproductive system, menopause affects several other aspects of a woman's health. One significant area is bone health. Estrogen plays a key role in maintaining bone density, and the decline in estrogen during menopause can contribute to bone loss, increasing the risk of osteoporosis and fractures.

Moreover, hormonal changes during menopause can influence metabolism and lead to weight gain, particularly around the abdomen. This shift in fat distribution is not only a cosmetic concern but also a health risk, as abdominal fat is associated with an increased risk of cardiovascular diseases.

Cognitive function may also be impacted during menopause, with some women reporting difficulties with memory and concentration.

This phenomenon, often referred to as "brain fog" is believed to be linked to hormonal fluctuations affecting the brain's neurotransmitters.

Emotionally, menopause can bring about mood swings, anxiety, and even symptoms of depression in some individuals. Hormonal changes can influence neurotransmitters like serotonin and dopamine, which play roles in regulating mood and emotional well-being.

While menopause is a natural and inevitable part of a woman's navigating impact on the body is complex and multifaceted.

Understanding these changes is crucial for women to navigate this phase with knowledge and proactive health measures. Embracing a holistic approach that includes a balanced diet, regular exercise, and emotional well-being strategies can contribute to a smoother transition and overall better quality of life during and after menopause.

Weight Issues in Menopause

Weight management becomes a significant concern for many women as they go through the intricate hormonal changes associated with menopause. The hormonal fluctuations, particularly the decline in estrogen levels, can contribute to shifts in metabolism and body composition, making weight management more challenging during this life stage.

One of the primary factors influencing weight gain during menopause is the redistribution of fat, commonly observed around the abdominal area.

This change in fat distribution is not merely a cosmetic issue; it has health implications. Abdominal fat, known as visceral fat, is metabolically active and has been linked to an increased risk of cardiovascular diseases, insulin resistance, and metabolic syndrome.

The decline in estrogen also plays a role in slowing down metabolism, making it easier for women to gain weight, especially if dietary and exercise habits remain unchanged.

Moreover, hormonal changes can affect insulin sensitivity, potentially leading to an increased likelihood of developing type 2 diabetes.

Emotional factors can further complicate weight management during menopause.

Mood swings, stress, and anxiety, which are common during this phase, may contribute to emotional eating or unhealthy dietary choices. Emotional well-being is intricately connected to eating habits, and addressing these psychological aspects is crucial in managing weight effectively.

To tackle weight issues during menopause, adopting a holistic approach is essential. A balanced and nutritious diet that prioritizes whole foods, lean proteins, and ample fruits and vegetables can support overall health and weight management.

Regular physical activity, including both cardiovascular exercises and strength training, is vital for boosting metabolism, maintaining muscle mass, and supporting weight loss.

for dietary and exercise considerations, managing stress and prioritizing mental health are integral components of a successful weight management strategy during menopause. Stress-reducing activities such as meditation, engaging in hobbies can positively impact both emotional well-being and weight.

It's important to note that each woman's experience during menopause is unique, and there is no one-size-fits-all solution to weight management. Consulting with healthcare professionals is the best choice.

CHAPTER 2: MENSTRATION AND ATHLETIC IMPACT

During menopause, certain health problems develop, and one area that attracts attention is the association between the menstrual cycle and sports performance.

The menstrual cycle is a complicated interplay of hormonal changes that may affect different physiological and psychological elements of a woman's body, and athletes, in particular, may suffer special obstacles.

The menstrual cycle is separated into various stages, notably the menstrual phase, follicular phase, ovulatory phase, and luteal phase. Each phase is marked by changes in hormone levels, with estrogen and progesterone playing major roles.

These hormones not only govern the reproductive system but also exert effects on energy consumption, thermoregulation, and neuromuscular function.

The menstrual cycle's possible influence on sports performance has been a topic of considerable attention and investigation. The menstrual phase, distinguished by the removal of the uterine lining and normally lasting approximately 3-7 days, may correlate with symptoms of exhaustion and reduced energy levels. Athletes may notice that they are weak in strength, endurance, and recuperation during this period.

The period of menstruation displays growing estrogen levels. This phase is often connected with higher energy and enhanced workout performance. Some athletes may discover that they enjoy greater strength and stamina during this period.

The ovulatory phase, occurring around the middle of the menstrual cycle, is distinguished by the release of an egg from the ovary. Estrogen levels peak during this time, perhaps favorably impacting athletic performance. Coordination, response time, and muscular function may be optimized.

The luteal phase, which occurs in the later part of the menstrual cycle, is marked by high progesterone levels. Some athletes may experience higher perceived effort during exercise, presumably owing to alterations in heat tolerance and fluid balance.

It's vital to highlight that individual variances occur, and not all women will experience these performance changes in the same manner. Factors such as exercise level, general health, and individual reactions to hormone changes contribute to the heterogeneity was seen.

Athletes facing menopause need to be alert to their bodies and alter training routines appropriately.

Understanding the connection between hormonal changes and athletic performance may enable women to maximize training tactics, manage recuperation efficiently, and handle unique issues connected with the menstrual cycle.

Developing open debate and knowledge regarding these concerns within the sporting community is vital.

Coaches, trainers, and athletes may work to develop support throughout that acknowledges the special requirements of female athletes throughout menopause, supporting a holistic approach to health and performance enhancement.

Athletes and Menopause

Changes in Metabolism and Energy Levels

Menopause frequently involves adjustments in metabolism and energy levels. This portion investigates how these changes might affect an athlete's stamina, endurance, and general energy management. Practical suggestions for modifying diet and exercise habits to support these changes are presented.

Hormonal Shifts and Their Effects on Physical Activity

Understanding the hormonal changes during menopause is vital for athletes. This section elucidates the function of estrogen, progesterone, and other hormones in the context of physical performance.

By appreciating these alterations, active women may better manage and enhance their training routines.

Obstacles and Strategies for Active Women

Navigating Emotional Changes and Body Image Challenges.

Beyond the physical changes, menopause may also influence mental well-being and body image. The psychological components of the menopausal journey, including ideas for controlling mood swings, increasing self-esteem, and promoting a good body image for active women.

Strategies for Active Women

Adapting workout programs to fit with the physiological changes during menopause is vital. Get practical ways for customizing exercises, ensuring they stay effective and supportive of overall well-being.

Overcome density pause-Related Obstacles

Building psychological resilience is vital for active women managing the difficulties of menopause, overcome challenges, manage stress, and build a resilient mentality that promotes sports performance and general life happiness.

This thorough investigation of menopause and its influence on active women goes beyond the scientific elements, giving concrete ideas and solutions to encourage women to flourish in their athletic endeavors throughout this transforming time of life.

Bone Health and Injury Prevention During Menopause

Menopause brings about considerable changes in a woman's hormonal landscape, and these changes may have a noteworthy influence on bone health. Estrogen, a hormone generated in the ovaries, plays a key function in maintaining bone density.

As estrogen levels fall throughout menopause, women become more prone to bone loss, leading to illnesses such as osteoporosis and an increased risk of fractures.

Osteoporosis is characterized by weaker and porous bones, rendering them more prone to fractures. The spine, hips, and wrists are typical locations of osteoporotic fractures, and the effects may be severe, limiting mobility and general quality of life.

To limit the risks associated with bone health after menopause, it is vital to implement techniques that enhance bone density and lower the incidence of injuries.

Regular weight-bearing workouts, such as walking, running, or resistance training is vital for maintaining bone density and strength. Weight-bearing activities stimulate bone-forming cells, helping to prevent the normal reduction in bone density that comes with aging and hormonal changes.

Appropriate calcium and vitamin D consumption is crucial for bone health. Calcium is a critical building component for bones, and vitamin D is important for the absorption of calcium.

Women experiencing menopause should ensure they acquire appropriate levels of essential nutrients via a balanced diet or supplements if required.

CHAPTER 3: NUTRITION

Athletes Nutritional Needs

Menopause triggers metabolic and hormonal changes, necessitating a reassessment of nutritional requirements.

The essential nutrients crucial for women athletes during this phase. Proteins, essential fats, complex carbohydrates, and micronutrients for their roles in supporting energy levels, muscle health, and overall well-being.

Hormone-Regulating Foods

Certain foods can positively impact hormonal balance. This part explores the incorporation of hormone-regulating foods into the diet.

Examples include foods rich in omega-3 fatty acids, antioxidants, and phytoestrogens. The discussion emphasizes the potential benefits of these foods in managing menopausal symptoms and optimizing athletic performance.

Hydration Strategies for Optimal Performance

Understanding Hydration Needs During Menopause

Menopausal changes influence hydration requirements. This section examines the importance of hydration, considering the impact of hormonal fluctuations on fluid balance.

Practical guidelines to help women athletes stay adequately hydrated, emphasizing the importance of regular water intake and monitoring individual hydration needs.

Electrolyte Balance and Menopause

Electrolytes play a crucial role in maintaining proper hydration and supporting muscle function. This part explores how hormonal changes during menopause can affect electrolyte balance.

Examples of electrolyte-rich foods are discussed, along with strategies for ensuring optimal levels through dietary choices and hydration practices.

Strategies for Hydration Timing

Timing of hydration significantly impacts athletic performance. Get a plan for timing fluid intake. Recommendations include pre- and post-exercise hydration, as well as consistent fluid intake throughout the day

Balancing Macronutrients

This section explores how meal composition can impact hormonal balance during menopause. Practical insights provided on achieving an optimal balance of carbohydrates, proteins, and fats to support hormonal health.

Examples include incorporating whole grains, lean proteins, and healthy fats into meals to provide sustained energy and support overall well-being.

Incorporating Anti-Inflammatory Foods

Inflammation can impact performance and recovery. The chapter discusses the role of inflammation during menopause and suggests incorporating anti-inflammatory foods into the diet. Examples include fruits, vegetables, and omega-3 rich foods, offering practical suggestions for integrating these foods into meals omega-3-richthletic performance.

Special Considerations for Menopausal healthy athletes

Metabolic shifts during menopause influence nutrient processing. This part offers tailored nutritional strategies to adapt to these changes.

Recommendations include adjusting calorie intake to account for changes in metabolism, ensuring menopausal athletes receive the necessary nutrients to support energy needs, and maintaining muscle, mass.

Weight Management and Body Composition

Menopause often coincides with changes in weight and body composition. This section guides maintaining a healthy body and body composition through proper nutrition. Practical advice includes portion control, mindful eating, and making nutrient-dense food choices to support fitness goals during menopause.

Meal Plans and Recipes

This section provides practical application by presenting sample meal plans tailored specifically for menopausal athletes. Meal plans include a balance of macronutrients, and incorporate hormone-regulating for <u>body</u> consider hydration needs. These exact simples offer tangible guidance for combining required nutrients into a regular diet.

To make nutritional guidance actionable, a collection of nutrient-rich recipes is needed. These recipes not only support hormonal balance and hydration but also cater to the taste preferences of active women.

Examples include meals that incorporate a variety of nutrient-dense ingredients, promoting overall well-being and enjoyment of a reconsidered during menopause.

Adjusting Diets to Hormonal Changes

Women suffer considerable hormonal fluctuations during menopause, which may drastically influence their dietary demands and metabolism. Understanding these changes is vital for developing a diet that successfully supports their health and performance.

Declining Estrogen Levels and Implications

A feature of menopause is the fall in estrogen production, a hormone that plays a crucial role in several ways biological processes, including: Bone health: Estrogen helps maintain bone mineral density, and its loss raises the risk of osteoporosis.

Body composition: Estrogen helps control fat distribution, and its reduction may lead to increasing body fat, especially around necessary.

Metabolism: Estrogen making insulin sensitivity and its loss may raise the risk of insulin resistance and type 2 diabetes.

Nutritional Strategies to Counteract Estrogen Decline

Increase calcium and vitamin D intake: These nutrients are necessary for sustaining bone health. Aim for 1,000-1,200 mg of calcium and 600-800 IU of vitamin D daily.

Prioritize protein intake: Protein is vital for muscle health and regeneration, which becomes even more critical after menopause. Aim for 1.2-1.6 grams of protein per kilogram of body weight daily.

Choose healthy fats: Include sources of omega-3 fatty acids, such as fatty fish, flaxseeds, and walnuts, which may enhance insulin sensitivity and vitamin ease inflammation.

Moderate carbohydrate intake: Focus on complex carbs from whole grains, fruits, and vegetables, which give sustained energy and fiber.

Limit processed meals and additional sugars: These foods may lead to weight gain and metabolic disorders.

Managing Energy Balance and Metabolism

Menopause frequently causes changes in energy balance and metabolism, making it hard to maintain a healthy weight or body composition. Tailoring calorie intake and macronutrient distribution is critical for controlling these changes.

Energy Balance and Menopause

During menopause, women's basal metabolic rate (BMR), the rate However they burn calories at rest, tends to drop. This makes it simpler to gain weight but harder to remove it.

Balancing and Expenditure

To maintain a healthy weight, modify calorie intake to reflect the lowered BMR. However, continue to participate in regular physical exercise, since it helps prevent the reduction in metabolism and increases lean muscle mass.

Optimizing Macronutrient Distribution

Protein: Prioritize protein consumption to maintain muscle mass and assist recovery after activity. Include high-quality protein sources such as lean meats, fish, eggs, lentils, and dairy.

Carbohydrates: Choose complex carbs from whole grains, fruits, and vegetables, which give sustained energy and fiber.

Healthy Fats: Include sources of omega-3 fatty acids, such as fatty fish, flaxseeds, and walnuts, which may enhance but harder and decrease inflammation.

Dietary customization is necessary for women athletes throughout menopause to maximize their nutrition and maintain their health and performance.

By recognizing the hormonal changes that occur during menopause and changing their meals appropriately, women may efficiently control their energy balance, metabolism, and body composition, while continuing to succeed in their athletic interests

Pre-Workout Nutrition Strategies

Pre-workout nutrition is crucial for menopausal athletes since it directly affects energy levels, attention, and general performance during activity.

With the background of hormonal changes, it becomes vital to feed the body with the correct nourishment. The emphasis is on ingesting a balanced meal combining carbs, proteins, and lipids to guarantee prolonged energy release and muscular support.

Strategic Macronutrient Distribution

Menopausal athletes benefit from a judicious allocation of macronutrients in their pre-workout meals. Carbohydrates serve as the major energy source, proteins promote muscular function, and healthy fats add to sustained energy. Examples include a balanced breakfast with whole grains, lean proteins, and healthy fats, giving a firm basis for future physical activities.

Hydration Strategies Before Exercise

Hydration is a core part of pre-workout preparation. Dehydration may impede performance, and hormonal changes during menopause might alter fluid balance.

Practical recommendations include proper water consumption and integrating hydrating meals such as water-rich fruits. Optimizing hydration before exercise ensures that menopausal athletes are well-prepared for optimum performance.

Post-Workout Recovery

Post-workout nutrition is a vital element of rehabilitation, especially for menopausal athletes. For its relevance in enabling muscle regeneration, restoring glycogen storage, and aiding overall recovery, supplying the body with the nutrients it needs for effective recovery after exercise.

Optimal Nutrient Timing for Recovery

Timing plays a significant role in post-workout nutrition. Menopausal athletes are educated on the ideal time for taking post-workout meals and snacks.

The focus is on the post-exercise window when the body is ready for nutritional absorption. Practical instructions guarantee that women may make educated decisions to optimize the advantages of post-workout nutrition.

Protein Synthesis and Muscle Repair

Protein is a vital component of post-workout recovery, promoting muscle synthesis and repair.

This segment goes into measures for maintaining enough protein consumption, including the selection of protein sources, portion sizes, and possible supplement usage.

Practical examples, such as a protein-rich supper with lean meats or plant-based proteins highlight effective approaches to boost muscle repair.

Balancing Carbohydrates for Glycogen Replenishment

Carbohydrates serve a critical function in restoring glycogen levels after exercise. This addresses the relevance of carbohydrates in the post-workout phase, offering insights into the kinds and quantities that enable glycogen restoration. Recommendations assist women in creating a balance that matches their training demands and menopausal concerns.

Hydration Strategies for Effective Recovery

Hydration remains a critical concern in the post-workout session. The chapter examines hydration measures for efficient recovery, highlighting the necessity of rehydration, maintaining electrolyte balance, and including hydrating meals. Practical advice aids women in maximizing their post-exercise hydration regimens, boosting total recovery.

By implementing these practical tactics for pre-workout nutrition and post-workout recovery, menopausal athletes may boost their exercise performance, assist their bodies in the recovery process and negotiate the particular challenges given by the menopausal transition

Nutritional and Diet Considerations

Nutrition has a vital role in promoting overall health during menopause, going beyond bone health to embrace a variety of physiological and psychological elements. A well-balanced diet may help control weight, promote hormonal balance, and ease some of the symptoms associated with menopause.

1. Calcium-Rich Foods: Dairy products, leafy green vegetables, and fortified meals are great sources of calcium. Incorporating them into everyday diets helps improve bone health.

2. Vitamin D Sources: Exposure to sunshine is a natural method to absorb vitamin D, although dietary sources including fatty fish,

fortified dairy products, and supplements may help to maintain health levels.

3. Protein Crucial: Protein is crucial for muscular health, and preserving muscle mass becomes particularly vital throughout menopause. Include lean sources of protein, such as chicken, fish, beans, and tofu, in your diet.

4. Whole Grains and Fiber: These help general digestive health and may assist in weight control, which is typically a problem during menopause.

5. Hydration: Staying appropriately hydrated is vital for several physical processes, including

through. Water enhances general well-being and may help ease symptoms like bloating.

6. Limiting Process Foods: Minimizing the consumption of processed foods, sweets, and excessive caffeine may help to improve hormonal balance and symptom management.

7. Balanced Nutrition: Prioritize a well-balanced diet rich in whole foods, including fruits, vegetables, whole grains, lean meats, and healthy fats. This supplies critical nutrients to support your shifting hormonal environment.

8. Healthy Fats: Include sources of healthy fats, such as avocados, almonds, and olive oil. These may contribute to hormone production and assist in regulating weight.

9. Limit Processed Foods: Minimize processed foods, refined sugars, and excessive caffeine, since they may worsen hormonal imbalances and lead to symptoms like hot flashes.

Adopting the best strategy that incorporates regular exercise, a nutrient-rich diet, and lifestyle adjustments are vital for preserving bone health and general well-being throughout menopause.

Women going through this era should engage closely with healthcare experts to build individualized solutions.

CHAPTER 4: EXERCISE PLAN FOR 30 DAYS

Weeks 1-2

Establishing a Foundation

- Day 1-5: Begin with low-impact workouts such as walking, swimming, or cycling for 30 minutes. Focus on developing a routine.

- Day 6-7: Incorporate modest strength training using bodyweight movements. Include squats, lunges, and push-ups.

- Day 8-14: Increase cardiac intensity by implementing interval training.

Alternate between periods of high and moderate intensity throughout your cardio activities.

- Day 15-21: Introduce more rigorous strength workouts. Include resistance exercise with dumbbells or resistance bands.

Weeks 3-4

Specialized Workouts

- Day 22-28: Explore exercises that increase flexibility and balance, such as yoga or Pilates. These may be especially effective during menopause.

- Day 29-30: Combine aerobic, strength, and flexibility exercises for a thorough workout. Consider a high-intensity interval training (HIIT) session for an efficient and productive exercise.

- Listen to Your Body: Pay attention to how your body reacts to various activities. Modify exercises as appropriate and allow for optimal recuperation.

- Stay Consistent: Consistency is crucial. Aim for at least 150 minutes of moderate-intensity aerobic activity each week, coupled with strength training activities at least twice a week.

- Include Rest Days: Allow your body time to rest and recuperate. Rest days are crucial to avoid overtraining and improve general well-being.

Remember, every woman's experience with menopause is unique. Adjust the intensity and kind of exercise depending on your fitness level and any pre-existing health concerns.

Combining a supportive diet and a well-structured fitness regimen, may assist greatly to managing the problems of menopause and fostering a healthy, active lifestyle.

CHAPTER 5: MENOPAUSE AND PHYSICAL HEALTH

Menopause is a crucial milestone in a woman's life, followed by hormonal upheavals that might impair physical health.

Crafting a conscious approach to diet becomes crucial during this period, comprising both items to avoid and a well-curated menopausal food list.

Foods to Avoid

1. Processed and Sugary Foods: High quantities of refined sugars might worsen symptoms such as mood swings and hot flashes. Minimize the intake of candy, pastries, and sugary drinks.

2. Caffeine: While moderate caffeine use is normally appropriate, excessive caffeine may lead to irritation and sleep difficulties. Consider minimizing coffee, tea, and energy drinks, particularly in the evening.

3. Salty Foods: Excess salt may lead to bloating and water retention, typical issues during menopause. Reduce consumption of processed meals and opt for fresh, natural foods to decrease salt levels.

4. Alcohol: Alcohol may disturb sleep patterns and lead to dehydration, which may worsen symptoms like hot flashes. Limit alcohol intake and keep well-hydrated.

5. Spicy Foods: For some women, spicy meals might provoke hot flashes and discomfort. Monitor your body's reaction and modify your spice consumption appropriately.

Foods to Eat

1. Calcium-Rich Foods: Strengthening bone health is vital throughout menopause. Incorporate dairy products, leafy greens, almonds, and fortified meals to maintain an appropriate calcium intake.

2. Fruits and Vegetables: Packed with critical vitamins, minerals, and antioxidants, fruits and vegetables contribute to overall health.

They may also aid in controlling weight, a typical worry during menopause.

3. Lean Proteins: Include sources of lean protein, such as chicken, fish, tofu, and lentils. Protein improves muscular health, which becomes particularly necessary when estrogen levels fall.

4. Healthy Fats: Go for sources of healthy fats, like avocados, nuts, seeds, and olive oil. These fats have a function in hormone synthesis and may assist in regulating weight.

5. Whole Grains: Choose whole grains like quinoa, brown rice, and oats. These give

sustained energy, fiber, and important nutrients.

6. Flaxseeds: Rich in omega-3 fatty acids, flaxseeds may help reduce symptoms like joint discomfort and improve heart health.

7. Soy Products: Foods containing soy, such as tofu and soy milk, contain substances called phytoestrogens that may help ease certain menopausal symptoms.

8. Water: Staying well-hydrated is vital. Water promotes different biological systems and may help alleviate symptoms like bloating.

Tips

- o Mindful Eating: Pay attention to hunger and fullness signals. Mindful eating may help reduce overeating and prone healthier digestion.

- o Small, Frequent Meals: Go for smaller, more frequent meals to control energy levels and maybe decrease symptoms like mood swings and exhaustion.

- o Consult a Nutritionist: Consider talking with a nutritionist who can give individualized counsel based on our unique requirements and interests.

A balanced and careful approach to eating is a critical component of sustaining physical health throughout menopause.

By being attentive to what you eat and adopting a range of nutrient-dense foods, you can assist your body during this transition period, minimizing symptoms and encouraging overall well-being.

Diet to Lose Belly Fat

As women reach menopause, hormonal changes generally lead to variations in body composition, with an increased propensity to retain fat in the abdominal area. Adopting a menopausal diet customized to suit this difficulty may be crucial in controlling weight and maintaining

> Balanced Caloric Intake: While lowering total calorie consumption may be important for weight control, excessive caloric restriction might be harmful. Focus on a balanced diet that fits your nutrition overcoming demands

> Emphasize Lean Proteins: Prioritize lean protein sources such as fish, chicken, tofu, and lentils. Protein is vital for maintaining muscular mass, which may assist in overcoming the normal drop in metabolism after menopause.

➢ Healthy Fats: Include sources of healthy fats including avocados, almonds, and olive oil. These fats contribute to fullness and may aid in regulating cravings.

➢ Whole Grains and Fiber: opt for whole grains like quinoa, brown rice, and oats, as well as fiber-rich dishes. Fiber stimulates digestion and might help you feel fuller for longer durations.

➢ Limit Added Sugars: Minimize the intake of sugary meals and drinks, since excess sugar might lead to belly fat buildup. Check food labels for hidden sugars.

➢ Hydration: Drink lots of water throughout the day. Staying well-hydrated boosts metabolism and may help reduce hunger.

➢ Regular Physical Activity: Combine a balanced diet with frequent exercise, including both cardiovascular activity and strength training. Exercise is vital for burning calories and preserving muscular mass.

Diet to Balance Hormones

✓ Phytoestrogen-Rich Foods: Incorporate foods containing phytoestrogens, such as soy products, flaxseeds, and whole grains. Phytoestrogens imitate the actions of estrogen in the body and may help regulate hormone levels.

✓ Omega-3 Fatty Acids: Include fatty fish, flaxseeds, chia seeds, and walnuts in your diet. Omega-3 fatty acids may help to hormonal balance and have anti-inflammatory qualities.

✓ Colorful Vegetables and Fruits: Consume a range of colorful vegetables and fruits high in antioxidants. These nutrients enhance general health and may help decrease oxidative stress linked with hormonal fluctuations.

✓ Avoid Endocrine Disruptors: Minimize exposure to endocrine-disrupting chemicals found in certain plastics, insecticides, and personal care items. These chemicals may interfere with hormone function.

✓ Manage Stress: Chronic stress may influence hormone levels. Incorporate stress-reducing methods such as meditation, yoga, or deep breathing exercises into your regimen.

✓ Adequate Sleep: Ensure you receive adequate quality sleep. Sleep is critical for hormonal homeostasis, and changes in sleep patterns may influence hormone balance.

✓ Regular Meals: Aim for frequent, balanced meals throughout the day. Irregular eating habits and missing meals might lead to hormone disorders.

Menopause and Vegetarian Diet

Menopause, a natural change in a woman's life, signifies the end of her reproductive years and is marked by a fall in estrogen and progesterone levels.

This hormonal transition brings to a range of physical and mental changes, including hot flashes, nocturnal sweats, mood swings, and changes in body composition.

For women adopting a vegetarian diet, menopause might provide extra nutritional concerns. As estrogen levels decline, the body's absorption and use of certain minerals, including as calcium, iron, and vitamin D, may be impaired.

To guarantee appropriate consumption of these vital nutrients and promote general health during menopause, consider the following dietary changes:

Calcium-Rich Foods: Adequate calcium consumption is critical for maintaining bone health, particularly during menopause when bone mineral density diminishes.

Include calcium-rich plant-based foods including fortified plant milks, tofu, leafy green vegetables, and calcium-set alginate. These alternatives offer a decent amount of calcium without the cholesterol and saturated fats frequently present in dairy products.

2. Iron-Rich Foods: Iron is vital for delivering oxygen throughout the body, and its shortage may lead to anemia. Include iron-rich plant-based meals such beans, lentils, fortified cereals, and dark leafy greens. Pair these meals with vitamin C-rich sources like citrus fruits and bell peppers to increase iron absorption.

3. Vitamin D-Rich Sources: Vitamin D serves a key function in calcium absorption and bone health. While the body may create vitamin D from sunshine exposure, it's vital to add dietary sources, particularly after menopause.

Include vitamin D-fortified plant milks, fatty fish (for non-vegan vegetarians), and mushrooms that have been exposed to sunshine. These options provide a plant-based strategy to acquiring vitamin D, which is typically restricted in vegetarian diets.

4. Phytoestrogens: Phytoestrogens are plant chemicals that have a similar

structure to estrogen and may help ease menopausal symptoms. Include phytoestrogen-rich foods like tofu, soy products, flaxseeds, and sesame seeds in your diet.

These plant-based estrogens may give a natural alternative to control menopausal symptoms without depending on hormone replacement treatment.

5. Whole Grains: Whole grains are a strong source of fiber, which may assist in digestion, control blood sugar levels, and support a healthy weight. Choose whole-grain bread, pasta, and cereals over refined substitutes. Whole grains include critical minerals and

fiber, which may help manage typical menopause-related symptoms including digestive difficulties and weight gain.

6. Fruits and Vegetables: Fruits and vegetables are rich with critical vitamins, minerals, and fiber, which are crucial for general health and well-being throughout menopause. Aim for a range of colored fruits and vegetables to increase nutritional intake.

Fruits and vegetables contain a varied variety of nutrients that promote overall health and may help minimize menopause-associated symptoms like weariness and skin dryness.

7. Limited Processed Foods and Added Sugars: Processed meals and added sugars may lead to weight gain, metabolic dysfunction, and inflammation, which can aggravate menopausal symptoms. Limit intake of these goods and opt for complete, unprocessed meals wherever feasible.

Minimizing processed foods and added sugars may help maintain a healthy weight, minimize inflammation, and enhance general health during menopause.

8. Hydration: Adequate water consumption is vital for general health and may help decrease menopausal symptoms like hot flashes and constipation. Aim for 8-10 glasses of water every day. Staying hydrated may help regulate

body temperature, avoid dehydration, and perhaps lower the frequency and severity of hot flashes.

Considerations

1. Consult a Registered Dietitian: A trained dietitian can give specialized nutrition advice to help you build a menopause-friendly vegetarian diet that suits your unique requirements and interests.

   Working with a licensed dietitian helps ensure you are fulfilling your nutritional needs and making smart food choices matched with your health objectives.

2. **Consider Supplements:** If dietary consumption of certain nutrients is insufficient, consider taking supplements, such as calcium, iron, and vitamin D. However, ask your doctor before taking any new supplements.

Supplements may be important to bridge any vitamin gaps in your diet, particularly if you have any underlying health issues that nutrient absorption maintaining Physical Activity: Regular exercise, especially weight-bearing activities, may assist maintain bone health, control

CHAPTER 6. MENTAL AND EMOTIONAL WELL-BEING

Menopause comprises not just physical changes but also major modifications in mental and emotional well-being.

Managing the emotional landscape throughout this transforming time is vital for a happy and empowered experience

1. Mindfulness Practices: - Integrate mindfulness practices into your routine. Mindful breathing, meditation, or yoga may help focus your mind, decrease stress, and boost overall emotional well-being.

2. Emotional Expression: - Acknowledge and express your feelings. Whether by writing,

chatting with a friend, or seeking professional therapy, allowing yourself to process and articulate your thoughts is crucial.

3. Social Connection: - Cultivate strong social relationships. Engage with friends, family, or support groups. Sharing experiences and emotions may generate a sense of camaraderie and understanding.

4. Positive Affirmations: - Incorporate positive affirmations into your everyday life. Affirmations may assist in transforming your mentality, boosting optimism and self-empowerment.

5. Self-Care Rituals: - Prioritize self-care activities. Whether it's a calming bath, a peaceful stroll in thoughts engaging in a cherished activity, these routines contribute to emotional well-being.

6. Professional Support: - Consider seeking the assistance of a mental health professional. A therapist or counselor may give essential insights, coping skills, and a secure environment for addressing emotional issues.

7. Thankfulness Practice: - Cultivate a thankfulness mentality. Regularly noticing and appreciating good parts of your life helps boost emotional resilience and attitude.

8. Embrace Change: - Menopause brings about considerable changes and mentally. Embrace this transformation with a positive perspective, considering it as a chance for personal progress and self-discovery.

9. Stress Reduction methods: - Practice stress reduction methods such as deep breathing, progressive muscle relaxation, or guided visualization. These approaches may assist in regulating stress levels and creating emotional equilibrium.

10. in regulating Lifestyle Habits: - Adopt overall healthy lifestyle habits, including frequent exercise, dieting, and adequate sleep. Physical well-being contributes considerably to mental and emotional resiliency.

11. Emotional Intelligence: - Develop emotional intelligence by understanding and

controlling your own emotions. Recognize and sympathize with the feelings of others, establishing stronger relationships.

12. Goal Setting: - Set reasonable and attainable objectives. Breaking major tasks into smaller, attainable stages may create a feeling of success and increase confidence.

Mental and emotional well-being is a dynamic and unique journey. What works for one individual may vary for another, be gentle with yourself as you negotiate the emotional terrain of menopause.

Seeking help and remaining alert to your mental health is a proactive step towards a more joyful and fulfilled menopausal experience.

CONCLUSION

As we end this comprehensive guide on menopause, it is our sincere hope that the information and insights shared empower you with the knowledge and tools to navigate this transformative phase with resilience, wellness, and wisdom.

Menopause is a natural and inevitable part of a woman's journey, and embracing it with a holistic approach can lead to a fulfilling and empowered experience.

Throughout this book, we've explored various facets of menopause, ranging from the physical changes and challenges to the nuanced aspects of mental and emotional well-being.

Understanding the hormonal shifts, adopting a balanced diet, engaging in regular exercise, and prioritizing self-care are integral components of a holistic approach to menopause.

The intricacies of menopause extend beyond the biological changes, encompassing the emotional and mental dimensions.

Strategies for managing stress, fostering positive emotions, and seeking support have been discussed to promote a comprehensive understanding of well-being during this period of transition.

We've got into specific topics such as bone health, athletic performance, and the impact of a vegetarian diet, recognizing that individual experiences are varied. Tailoring your approach to menopause based on your unique needs and preferences is essential, and seeking guidance from healthcare professionals ensures a personalized and informed journey.

Weight management, a common concern during menopause, has been addressed with practical tips, dietary considerations, and exercise plans designed to support your physical health and overall wellness.

The interconnected nature of physical and mental well-being has been emphasized, reinforcing the importance of a holistic lifestyle approach.

As you move forward, remember that menopause is not a one-size-fits-all experience. Your journey is uniquely yours, and embracing this transition with grace and self-compassion is key.

Seek support from healthcare professionals, engage in open conversations with loved ones, and celebrate the wisdom that comes with this life chapter.

May this guide serve as a companion on your menopausal journey, offering insights, encouragement, and practical strategies for embracing the changes while maintaining a sense of vitality and well-being.

Navigate menopause with wellness, wisdom, and a resilient spirit, ushering in a new chapter of life with grace and strength.

BONUS

EXERCISE JOURNAL

Training Focus

CARDIO

Exercise	Set	Rep	Heart Rate

STRENGTH TRAINING

Exercise	Set	Rep	Heart Rate

GOALS

NOTES

EXERCISE JOURNAL

Training Focus

CARDIO

Exercise	Set	Rep	Heart Rate

STRENGTH TRAINING

Exercise	Set	Rep	Heart Rate

GOALS

NOTES

EXERCISE JOURNAL

Training Focus

CARDIO

Exercise	Set	Rep	Heart Rate

STRENGTH TRAINING

Exercise	Set	Rep	Heart Rate

GOALS

NOTES

EXERCISE JOURNAL

Training Focus

CARDIO

Exercise	Set	Rep	Heart Rate

STRENGTH TRAINING

Exercise	Set	Rep	Heart Rate

GOALS

NOTES

EXERCISE JOURNAL

Training Focus

CARDIO

Exercise	Set	Rep	Heart Rate

STRENGTH TRAINING

Exercise	Set	Rep	Heart Rate

GOALS

NOTES

EXERCISE JOURNAL

Training Focus

CARDIO

Exercise	Set	Rep	Heart Rate

STRENGTH TRAINING

Exercise	Set	Rep	Heart Rate

GOALS

NOTES

EXERCISE JOURNAL

Training Focus

CARDIO

Exercise	Set	Rep	Heart Rate

STRENGTH TRAINING

Exercise	Set	Rep	Heart Rate

GOALS

NOTES

EXERCISE JOURNAL

Training Focus

CARDIO

Exercise	Set	Rep	Heart Rate

STRENGTH TRAINING

Exercise	Set	Rep	Heart Rate

GOALS

NOTES

EXERCISE JOURNAL

Training Focus

CARDIO

Exercise	Set	Rep	Heart Rate

STRENGTH TRAINING

Exercise	Set	Rep	Heart Rate

GOALS

NOTES

EXERCISE JOURNAL

Training Focus

CARDIO

Exercise	Set	Rep	Heart Rate

STRENGTH TRAINING

Exercise	Set	Rep	Heart Rate

GOALS

NOTES

EXERCISE JOURNAL

Training Focus

CARDIO

Exercise	Set	Rep	Heart Rate

STRENGTH TRAINING

Exercise	Set	Rep	Heart Rate

GOALS

NOTES

EXERCISE JOURNAL

Training Focus

CARDIO

Exercise	Set	Rep	Heart Rate

STRENGTH TRAINING

Exercise	Set	Rep	Heart Rate

GOALS

NOTES

EXERCISE JOURNAL

Training Focus

CARDIO

Exercise	Set	Rep	Heart Rate

STRENGTH TRAINING

Exercise	Set	Rep	Heart Rate

GOALS

NOTES

EXERCISE JOURNAL

Training Focus

CARDIO

Exercise	Set	Rep	Heart Rate

STRENGTH TRAINING

Exercise	Set	Rep	Heart Rate

GOALS

NOTES

EXERCISE JOURNAL

Training Focus

CARDIO

Exercise	Set	Rep	Heart Rate

STRENGTH TRAINING

Exercise	Set	Rep	Heart Rate

GOALS

NOTES

EXERCISE JOURNAL

Training Focus

CARDIO

Exercise	Set	Rep	Heart Rate

STRENGTH TRAINING

Exercise	Set	Rep	Heart Rate

GOALS

NOTES

EXERCISE JOURNAL

Training Focus

CARDIO

Exercise	Set	Rep	Heart Rate

STRENGTH TRAINING

Exercise	Set	Rep	Heart Rate

GOALS

NOTES

EXERCISE JOURNAL

Training Focus

CARDIO

Exercise	Set	Rep	Heart Rate

STRENGTH TRAINING

Exercise	Set	Rep	Heart Rate

GOALS

NOTES

EXERCISE JOURNAL

Training Focus

CARDIO

Exercise	Set	Rep	Heart Rate

STRENGTH TRAINING

Exercise	Set	Rep	Heart Rate

GOALS

NOTES

EXERCISE JOURNAL

Training Focus

CARDIO

Exercise	Set	Rep	Heart Rate

STRENGTH TRAINING

Exercise	Set	Rep	Heart Rate

GOALS

NOTES

EXERCISE JOURNAL

Training Focus

CARDIO

Exercise	Set	Rep	Heart Rate

STRENGTH TRAINING

Exercise	Set	Rep	Heart Rate

GOALS

NOTES

EXERCISE JOURNAL

Training Focus

CARDIO

Exercise	Set	Rep	Heart Rate

STRENGTH TRAINING

Exercise	Set	Rep	Heart Rate

GOALS

NOTES

www.ingramcontent.com/pod-product-compliance
Lightning Source LLC
Chambersburg PA
CBHW050737260726
48661CB00001B/283